Before CHiLDBiRTH

Before CHiLDBiRTH

Dr. Corinne Brosseau

Before Childbirth
First Edition 1990, Second Edition 1994

To order additional copies of this book, contact:
Xlibris Corporation
1-888-795-4274
www.Xlibris.com
Orders@Xlibris.com
71699

Contents

ACKNOWLEDGMENT & DEDICATION

I would like to acknowledge the Lord Jesus Christ who without Him and the Holy Spirit our child and book would have been totally impossible.

I dedicate this book to our daughter, Tiffany, who is such a happy, peaceful, joyful reward from the very throne room of God.

FOREWORD

"THIS BOOK TEACHES women how to speak the blessings of God over their unborn baby to ensure a healthy pregnancy and birth. Corinne shares prayers to pray over your baby that are found in the Bible which will cause God's amazing blessings to rest upon your child and His protection throughout your pregnancy. I highly recommend this book."

Dr. Steve Barry
Founder & Pastor
Christian Family Church International
Jupiter, Florida

INTRODUCTION

THE PURPOSE OF writing this book is to give glory to God and to share with you the blessings that His Word had for me and how you can have the same for your baby-to-be.

The word says that we overcome by the word of our testimony (Rev.12:11) . . . that is why I felt compelled to tell my story. After you read this book you will see that His word is true.

I can only say that I would not have wanted to be without the knowledge of His precious word during my pregnancy and childbirth. We are to choose life and not death. What we speak is what we believe and gives rise to our faith. I have found that by reading and acting upon God's word, and by confessing His truths, that I have a stronger faith. I know the gospel is the power of God unto salvation to everyone who believes (Rom. 1:16). Every promise of God contains the power of God to produce what it says when we choose to believe and do it. I pray that this book will bring many blessings to you.

I have had many people come and tell me that when I prayed the promises of God for them they had a very pleasant, fast, safe birthing of their little gift from God. God will do the same for you also.

My intent for writing this book was to be a tool or guide to help new parents to understand and acquire the blessings and rewards that

God has ordained for them to have, as promised in His written word and how to use them with prayers.

It is by no means a scientific research study but merely an example of how science has been found to line up with what God said was true all along. These promises are ours to appropriate for soundness of mind, without fear, and grounded in truth of His word. The truth will always set free the one who seeks and finds it (John 8:32).

CHAPTER ONE

DECREE A THING!

TWO KEYS TO know that as a covenant child of God you can be prepared for your pregnancy and can have a perfect baby. The bible says that *"You will also decree a thing, and it will be established for you;" (Job 22:28)*. "If you have been snared with the words of your mouth, have been caught with the words of your mouth. Do this, my son (or daughter), and deliver yourself" (Proverbs 6:2-3).

This means we are to say what God says about our baby. He says that there is power in our words. We can either say good things or bad things, but either way, they will have an effect, outcome, and consequence. This is not to be confused with 'positive' confession. You can confess something positively until you are blue in the face and it will not come to pass. What makes the powerful difference here is that you are confessing "His Word" NOT your own words. The bible says God made the worlds by the power of His spoken Word (Hebrews 11:3). Jesus told the apostles that if they had faith and did not doubt that they could *say* unto the mountain, be thou removed and cast into the sea and it would be done *(Matt. 21:21 KJV)*.

There is power in God's word and His promises for us. If we say what HE SAYS, we have that assurance that: *"So shall My word be which goes forth from My mouth; it shall not return to Me empty, without accomplishing what I desire and without succeeding in the matter for which I sent it"* (Isa. 55:11).

This is POWERFUL. This is His Promise to us. All we have to do to put it in motion is to *"say"* it with our mouth, believe it in our heart, and not doubt. The burden then remains upon God to uphold and perform His word. Every person I have known who has done this; (including myself and my family) who have confessed God's word over their baby from the beginning of conception have had wonderful, beautiful, healthy and blessed children. God will bless you beyond measure because you are doing what He said to do. The results will be that your joy will be so full that you will hardly be able to contain it. I have to say that from my own personal testimony too, I have been greatly blessed. My daughter has been a gift from God. She is such an instrument of joy and a true reward from Him, as He says in (Psalm 127: 3-5 AMP): *"Behold, children are a heritage from the Lord, the fruit of the womb a reward. As arrows are in the hand of a warrior, so are the children of one's youth. Happy, blessed and fortunate is the man whose quiver is filled with them."* I have to say that this is absolutely true. As Jesus would preface it "Truly, I say unto you . . ." (Matt. 24:34).

After being married for about three years [and also being forty-one years of age] my husband and I decided we wanted to have a child. I confessed: "I am *planted in the house of the Lord, we will flourish in the courts of our God. I will <u>still yield fruit in old age (not that forty-one is all that old)</u>: I shall be full . . . To declare that the Lord is upright"* (Psalm 92:13-15). I could not conceive prior to this decision but God did a special work in our lives and we became pregnant.

As I was in prayer one day I asked Him what we should name the baby and He gave me her name. It was to be *"manifestation of God"*. I looked up *"manifestation"* and I found *"theophany"* in my dictionary. "Theo" in Greek means God and *"phaneia"* means manifestation or appearance. I found a baby name book and it listed the translation of this to be *"epiphany"* and the English name is **"Tiffany"**.

". . . Even from the womb He has called me by that name"
(Isaiah 49:1).

It was through confessing God's word that we conceived and it was through the continuation of confessing His word over her in my womb that brought forth good fruit. I had a very relaxing pregnancy. I had slight morning sickness (maybe two or three times at the most) in the beginning, as this was my first child and I did not expect this to happen. So I promptly started confessing that my body would line up to the Word of God. After that, I had no further morning sickness. I had no pain during 24 hours after my water broke. During the whole 24 hour period after the water broke I confessed and had normal muscle contractions. Our daughter's heartbeat remained a steady 146 throughout the total pre-delivery time until birth. The doctor could not believe she had not stressed out during this long period; but I believe that it was God's unending favor, grace, our faith in the word, and prayers that were spoken over our baby for the past nine months that brought both of us through safely and with no problems. *"The Lord will perfect that which concerns me." (Psalms 138.8 AMP).*

Everything went smooth and we had a healthy baby, alert and full of joy, who is truly an instrument of joy and love, as well as a miracle baby. *Jesus said "Be it done unto you according to your faith"* (Matt. 9:29). Psalm 57.2 in *The Amplified Bible it reads:* "I will cry to the God Most High, Who performs on my behalf and rewards me – Who brings to pass His purposes for me and surely completes them." There was an inner peace the whole time, knowing that God was in control of this situation, and I believe I would never have conceived and delivered safely without the Word of God planted by our speaking His words over her.

We did not expect having a cesarean birth, but sometimes things do not work out the way we may plan them or think they should, but they **DO WORK** out for good to those who pray and are called according to His purpose! "For I know the plans I have for you, declares the Lord, 'plans for welfare and not for calamity to give you a future and a hope.' 'Then you will call upon Me and come and pray to Me, and I <u>will listen</u> to you . . .'" says the Lord (Jeremiah 29:11-12). "They overcame by the blood of the Lamb and the <u>word of their testimony.</u>" Emphasis added, (Rev. 12:11 KJV).

*   *   *

CHAPTER TWO

HIS WILL AND COVENANT WITH YOU

Y OUR BABY *IS* His will and covenant at work in you to work for His good pleasure. It is not up to us to produce – it's up to God because it is His own word! *"Know therefore that the Lord thy God, He is God; the faithful God which keepeth covenant and mercy with them that love Him and keep His commandments to a thousand generations" (Deut. 7:9). "For thou art an holy people unto the Lord thy God: the Lord thy God hath chosen thee to be a special people unto himself, above all the people that are upon the face of the earth" (Deut. 7:6 KJV).*

God had always had good plans in mind for us.

> *". . . He who began a good work in you, will continue until the day of Jesus Christ – right up until the time of His return, developing the good work, and perfecting and bringing it to full completion in you" (Phil. 1:6 AMP).*

We can have faith because what God says is true; He is at work within us both to will and to do his good pleasure (Phil. 2:13 KJV).

I can say from personal experience that everything He has promised has always been true. So then, we know that if He says He is at work in us we have confidence that He is working on behalf of our child also when we speak His promises for our new child.

> *"And this is the confidence which we have before Him, that, if we ask anything according to His will He hears us. And if we know that He hears us in whatever we ask we know that we have the request which we have asked from Him. (I John 5:14-15).*

> *The bible says in (Jeremiah 29: 11-12) words that give hope: "For I know the plans that I have for you, declares the Lord, 'plans for welfare and not for calamity to <u>give you</u> a future and a hope.' Then you will call upon Me and pray to Me, and I <u>will listen</u> to you . . ."' (Jer. 29:11-12).*

Your baby is part of God's covenant if you are a free woman, i.e., an heir of the promise through the seed of Abraham which is Christ [the Anointed One] Jesus. If you want to be sure you are a child of God and a partaker of His covenant you<u> must know beyond any shadow of a doubt</u> that you have the Gift of Eternal Life which makes you His child. If you would like to be sure, just say this short prayer from your heart . . . *"Father God, in the Name of Jesus Christ of Nazareth I come before you and confess with my mouth that I want to be forgiven of all my sins, that you would come into my heart and cleanse me of all unrighteousness and make me a child of God. Make me the person you ordained. Fill me with your Holy Spirit that I might know the power of your word for me to fulfill your good pleasure. Thank You Lord, that I have the Gift of Eternal Life; I am now a covenant child of yours, and an heir to your kingdom."*

Anyone who confesses with his mouth and believes in his heart, the Lord Jesus Christ, shall be saved (Acts 16:31). This means you will know beyond any doubt that you are His child and you have entered into eternal life. The apostle Paul says *"And you brethren, like Isaac, are children of promise"(Gal. 4:23). "But the son by the bond [slave] woman was born according to the flesh, and the son of the free woman [child of God] through the promise (Gal.4:23 KJV). (Emphasis added)*

IF IT IS HIS WILL, THEN HE WILL BRING IT TO PASS. IF HE FORMS YOUR BABY – HE/SHE WILL BE PERFECTLY MADE IN HIS IMAGE.

"Thus says the Lord who <u>made</u> you and <u>formed</u> you from the womb, who will <u>help</u> you" (Isa. 44:2).

"As for Me, this is My covenant or league with them, says the Lord: My Spirit, Who is upon you [and Who writes the law of God inwardly on the heart], and My words which I have put in your mouth shall not depart out of your mouth, or out of the mouths of your [true, spiritual] children, or out of the mouths of your children's children, says the Lord, from henceforth and forever" (Isa. 59:21 AMP).

Your baby is a spiritual blessing from God as it was <u>formed</u> from <u>before the foundation of the world.</u> *"Blessed be the God and Father of our Lord Jesus Christ, who has blessed us with every spiritual blessings in the heavenly places IN Christ just as He chose us in Him <u>before</u> the <u>foundation</u> of the world, that we should be holy and blameless before Him" (Ephesians 1:3-4).*

Prayers of Dedication

Father, I dedicate my baby to you and I say that it is written in your word that . . . *[You can substitute your baby's name in place of "my baby" when you pray this."]* we have Your grace and peace multiplied unto us through the knowledge of God, and of Jesus our Lord (2 Pet. 1:2 KJV).

The LORD will guard my baby's going out and coming in from this time forth and forever (Ps 121:8).

We have God who works in us, both to do his will and good pleasure (Phil 2:13 KJV).

* * *

CHAPTER THREE

A PERFECT BABY

GOD HAS TOLD us of our origin. That we were in His thoughts before He allowed us to come into existence. In Jeremiah, Chapter 1 it says he *knew us before* he formed us. His eyes beheld our unformed substance *[as an embryo]*. He had designed every part of us and wrote it down in His Book and then knit us together in our mother's womb.

> "For thou didst *form* my inward parts; Thou didst weave me in my mother's womb. I will give thanks to Thee, for I am *fearfully and wonderfully made;* Wonderful are Thy works, and my soul knows it very well. My frame was not *hidden* from Thee, when *I was made in secret, and skillfully wrought* in the depths of the earth. Thine eyes have seen my unformed substance; and in Thy book they were all written, the days that were ordained for me, when as yet there was not one of them" (Psalms 139: 13-15).

"For I am confident of this very thing, that He who began a good work in you will perfect it until the day of Christ Jesus" (Philippians 1:6). *God is saying it is okay to ask of Him, being our Father in Heaven, and He will give us good things (Matt. 7:7,11 KJV).*

JESUS FORMED YOUR BABY; THEREFORE IT IS POSITIONED PROPERLY: Before He formed me in the belly He knew me; and before I came out of the womb He sanctified me (Jer. 1:5, KJV).

"For I am His workmanship created in Christ Jesus for good works which God prepared beforehand, that we should walk in them" (Eph. 2:10).

THEREFORE YOUR SEED IS THE SEED HE CREATED WITHIN THE WOMB.

*   *   *

CHAPTER FOUR

POWER, LOVE, AND A SOUND MIND

F EAR IS A negative type of faith. To operate in fear means we are not operating in faith and God says that we please Him if we live by faith. The just shall live by faith.

> *"For God has not given us a spirit of fear; but of power, and of love, and of a sound mind" (2 Tim. 1:7 KJV).*

When God created Adam and Eve, He made Eve to bear children without pain. The pain did <u>not come upon</u> the human race until "the Fall" of Adam and Eve. (Genesis 3:16 KJV) states "*Unto the woman he said, I will greatly multiply thy sorrow and thy conception; in sorrow thou shalt bring forth children; and thy desire shall be to thy husband, and he shall rule over thee.* The definition of "sorrow" in Hebrew Old Testament text is `*itstsabown:* pain, labor, hardship, sorrow, and toil;[1] which came upon fallen man.

As part of that curse came fear and pain. When Christ came, he redeemed us from the curse of the law, being made a curse for us (Gal. 3:13-14). Therefore, we do not have to accept any part of that old curse which Satan will try to make us believe. (He wants to keep God's children in darkness and bondage as long as possible.)

When we walk by faith we say we do not accept what the world says (Jesus said Satan is the God of this world system), but that we accept what God's word says instead. By deciding to stand on the word and hold God to His promise we activate faith in our lives (I Tim.2:15).

Scientists are now finding out that pain is <u>NOT</u> a primary reflex reaction. Pain only comes secondary after we tell our brain that there should be pain. Teaching and education in this area are important. God says his people are destroyed for lack of knowledge (Hosea 4:6). When the brain is properly trained, new conditioned reflexes help the brain to handle the demands of childbirth.[2] The brain correlates conditioned signals that allow painless stimulus to become painful.[3] The other side of the coin is that if the brain has that kind of ability based on knowledge to allow pain upon the body, then why not reverse it, and use that power to bring forth the opposite – for example – endorphins. (Endorphins are a hormone excreted by the brain, which have an opium-type numbing effect on the body.) The point being, if God gave us power and a sound mind, then we should use it for good and train it like He says.

Research has proven that women who were educated in the area of childbirth, who knew what to expect and were prepared for it, along with relaxation and proper coaching, and <u>use of words</u>, experienced no pain.[4] Contractions are automatic, but God says we can speak the word to our situation and it will go forth and not return void. There is a connection here between the Word spoken and what was just discussed in regard to words. I believe therefore, that the pain *comes after* the brain tells the body to feel it. When a person allows fear to take over, that fear tells the brain how to react. God is telling us that <u>knowledge overrides fear</u> and enables one to be of sound mind (2 Tim. 1:7). Scientists say words and speech have a lot to do with this process and, as we know, this lines up exactly with the word of God. We can have what we say. *"Death and life are in the power of the tongue; and they that love it shall eat the fruit thereof" (Prov. 18:21 KJV)*.

What we say goes to our brain and is transmitted to the body. So, here we have secular science proving that what God says is true. When we believe by faith, and speak the word of God, we can expect to be free from the curse. As of 1955 statistics show 700,000 women in China, not to mention many in Asia, have given birth without pain, based simply upon man's knowledge.[5] God says about His children that they are destroyed for lack of knowledge" *(Hosea 4:6 KJV)*. Knowledge destroys fear, which in turn, I believe, helps us overcome pain.

If the world can use its soul-mentality to deliver themselves from pain, how much <u>more</u> can the child of God do so spiritually, as well as mentally?

We have been given the power by God to confess His word to our bodies, activate it by our faith, and rest in knowing that God is well able to perform all that he promised. We may not understand *how* God does it, but if we understand as much as we can about what he gave us (our bodies being a temple of the Holy Spirit) then He <u>will accomplish</u> the rest, as we are in covenant with Him. He will honor His word. The burden is on Him to perform, as He is not as a man that He should lie. If we reject the knowledge of God he says: *"Because thou hast rejected knowledge, I will also reject thee . . . seeing thou hast forgotten the law of thy God, I will also forget thy children" (Hosea 4:6 KJV)*.

If we confess the word we issue forth power: *"Death and life are in the power of the tongue: and they that love it shall eat the fruit thereof" (Prov. 18:21 KJV)*. It is easy to snare ourselves when we speak wrong words, and to get trapped by the belief of those wrong words (Prov. 6:2 KJV).

We have a choice – to speak life and blessing to our bodies and command any process to make it line up with what God says in the Name of Jesus Christ and it will bring victory; *or* we can choose death and speak what the world has told us to our bodies and babies. He says in Proverbs 3:8 *"Fear the Lord and turn away from evil. It will be healing to your body, and refreshment to your bones."* In Proverbs 4:22 His words are *"life to those who find them,* **and health to all their whole body.**"

*   *   *

End Notes:

[1]   Based on definition from <u>Strong's Greek/Hebrew Dictionary</u>, (Thomas Nelson Publishers) 1984, "sorrow" 6093.

Fernand Lamaze, <u>Painless Childbirth</u> (Henry Regnery Company) 1970, 117.

Ibid, 68.

Ibid, 32.

Ibid, 35.

Note: Although we are still subject to physical death (Rom. 8.2) because of the curse of the Fall on all of mankind (which causes our bodies to become slaves of sin and death), we can appropriate God's word as a born-again child of God and pass from spiritual death to spiritual life. We can walk in overcoming victory because the word says Jesus redeemed us (Gal. 3:13).

CHAPTER FIVE

NO FEAR – NO PAIN

MANY PEOPLE HAVE been taught through word of mouth that when they hear the word "contraction" it automatically means "pain". This is a fallacy. What we know through science has now been proven that people can be conditioned to expect pain.[1] By the same standard we can condition our brain to function the way we tell it if we have the proper teaching and training to do so. The first step is to understand what we are referring to here. To start with, let us take the word *"contract"*. One meaning is to draw together so as to become diminished in size, shrink, or deflate.[2] Therefore, to have contractions means a functioning muscle is in the process of contracting (i.e. the uterus shrinks in order to push the baby out). This process is a spontaneous, natural thrusting action of the uterus.

A famous French obstetrician, by the name of Lamaze, introduced breathing techniques for natural childbirth and delivery as well as other methods for preventing the occurrence of pain.[2]

Many women have gone to Lamaze classes to learn proper breathing techniques for their deliveries. When the technique is taught and coached there is a vast difference in the outcome. Remember, a contraction is when the uterus is shrinking in order to push the baby out. This process is a spontaneous, *natural action* of the uterus. There is no indication that there should be pain associated with this certain natural muscle action if the correct steps are taken to allow the brain to adapt and function.[2] God says his children are destroyed for lack of knowledge (Hosea 4:6). Therefore, for a muscle to contract can be done without pain once the fear is eliminated. Such pain would be secondary and caused more from *not* understanding and from fear, or having no control over the function of the body during this process. Everyone these days is familiar with what stress does to the body. Well, fear will bring on stress real fast. When a person is in fear they tense up. When the body is tense is experiences pain. This tenseness is a separate function not to be associated with contractions. "God did not give us a spirit of timidity – of cowardice, of craven and cringing and fawning fear – but He has given us a spirit of power, love and a calm and well-balanced mind, discipline, and self-control" (2 Tim 1:7 AMP). When we say this promise, out loud *(say above scripture verse using the "me" pronoun instead of "us")* faith starts to rise in us and the fear goes. I say this because during my twenty-four hours of contractions – what I experienced was not pain – work, but not pain.

Another well-known and also misquoted phrase is "labor pains". Many use the phrase "labor pains" to mean "muscle contractions" and vice versa. But the two are quite different, and cause a different response from the body.

During my muscle contractions and with proper breathing I was able to handle each one with a normal, calm control. I would hardly say that it was pain.

We need to confess with our mouth that we will have <u>muscle contractions,</u> (which is a natural function of the body created by God) and NOT <u>labor pains.</u> *"<u>Before</u> she travailed, she brought forth; <u>before</u> her pain came, she was delivered of a man child"* (Isaiah 66:7 KJV). Some fear many things: i.e., especially old wives tales, other's experiencing a certain age to bear children, etc. But what does God say: *"I will set him securely on high, with long life I will satisfy him"* (Psalm 91:16 KJV). *"They that are planted in the house of the Lord they flourish in the courts of our God. They will still yield fruit in old age: they shall be full of sap and very green. To declare that the Lord is upright. (Psalm 92: 13-15).*

God blesses us with children so He can get the glory for it. *"For I will contend with him who contends with you, and I will give safety to your children"* (Isaiah 49:25b AMP).

As a child of God you are in Christ and in Christ you have the anointing. The anointing is what breaks the yoke of bondage to the curse. In Christ [the Anointed One] we as children of God partake of that anointing. Jesus said *"Come to Me, all who are weary and heavy-laden, and I will give you rest. Take My yoke upon you, and learn from Me, for I am gentle and humble in heart; and you shall find rest for your souls. For My yoke is easy, and My load is light"* (Matthew 11: 28-30).

COVENANT WOMEN ARE NOT UNDER THE LAW OF SIN AND DEATH BUT UNDER THE SPIRIT OF LIFE IN CHRIST JESUS WHICH HAS SET US FREE.

> *"Christ hath redeemed us from the curse of the law, being made a curse for us"* (Gal. 3:13 KJV).

> *"For the law of the Spirit of Life in Christ Jesus hath made me free from the law of sin and death"* (Rom. 8:2 KJV).

Jesus used childbirth as an example to the apostles about sorrow and His leaving them when He said: *"Whenever a women is in travail (i.e., Grk: tikto – to produce, bear, bring forth or be delivered) she has* **sorrow, because her hour has come;** *but when she gives birth to the child, she remembers the anguish (i.e., Grk: thlipsis – burden or tribulation from that burden – to crowd, narrow) no more, for joy that a child has been born into the world"* (John 16:21).

I believe Jesus was explaining the feeling of sorrow of his leaving them not physical pain but a heartfelt pain and anguish of parting. *"Understanding is a fountain of life unto him that has it"* (Proverbs 16:22). *"Be it done unto you according to your faith"* (Matt. 9:29 KJV).

* * *

End Notes:

1   Fernand Lamaze, <u>Painless Childbirth</u> (Henry Regnery Company) 1970, p.68-69.

2   Based on definition <u>Webster's Collegiate Dictionary</u>, 10th ed., s.v. "contract".

3   Ibid, 68.

4   Ibid, 68-69.

CHAPTER SIX

SPEEDY PRE-DELIVERY and SAFE DELIVERY

AS A CHILD of God we are of the seed of Abraham and have the same blessings of the covenant that God had with his children in the old covenant and much more because we have a <u>greater covenant now</u> through the blood of Christ. *"And the midwives said to Pharaoh "Because the Hebrew women are not as the Egyptian women; for they are vigorous and they give birth before the midwife can get to them"* (Exodus 1:19).

Vigorous: i.e., from lively in Hebrew "CHAYAH" meaning to preserve, alive, life, to be whole.[1]

Remember the Hebrew women were under the Old Covenant, and they delivered speedily. How much more now as children of Abraham under the New Covenant can we expect for God to hold true to his promises with His covenant children. *"Now to Him who is able to do exceeding abundantly beyond all that we ask or think, according to the power that works WITHIN US"* (Eph. 3:20).

That POWER is the power of the promise given to us by God. When we speak the promise, God has to honor it because it is His own word of His covenant.

"Notwithstanding she shall be <u>saved</u> (i.e. Grk. renders to save, deliver or protect, heal, preserve, make whole. "SOZO") in childbearing, if they continue in faith and charity and holiness with sobriety" (I Tim. 2:15 KJV).

FACE-DOWN, HEAD-FIRST DELIVERY

GOD MAKES SURE HIS WILL IS DONE. JESUS IS THERE WITH YOU TO DELIVER YOUR BABY. *"He shall feed His flock like a shepherd: He shall gather the lambs with His arms, and carry them in His bosom, and shall gently lead those that are with young" (Isaiah 39:11KJV).*

Not only confessing but even singing. That's right – singing! Get caught up with singing; your whole spirit, soul and body unto God because the bible says God inhabits the *praises* of his people. His presence is there with the singing and the joy comes. The joy of the Lord brings with it a portion of faith. I believe God permeates the very atmosphere around us as praises to Him are sent out. How much more would He then be there to make sure your child would be delivered the way he ordained it from the beginning. God does say, *"Before she travailed, she brought forth; before her pain came, she gave birth . . ."*

A precious sister in the Lord who ministers in song has sung in the spirit many times during the birth of a little one and in a very short time the baby comes. With this type of atmosphere faith rises and fear dies. It is important to stay full of faith and not yield to negative thoughts. When you sing unto God, it is easy to stay centered on the truth and on His Word. The other side of the coin is to allow yourself to think negative thoughts and speak about negative situations. This opens the door to fear.

"You who have been borne by Me from birth and have been carried from the womb . . . I have done it, and I shall carry you and I shall bear you, and I shall deliver you" (Isaiah 46: 3-4).

"Yet thou art He who dist bring me forth from the womb" (Psalm 22:9). "Because he has loved Me, therefore I will deliver him" (Ps. 91:14).

"BEFORE, she travailed she brought forth; before her pain came, she gave birth to a boy (Isaiah 66:7). "Who has heard such a thing? Who has seen such things" . . . Shall I bring to the point of birth and not give delivery? says the Lord; shall I who gives delivery shut the womb? says your God" (Isaiah 66: 8-9).

CHILDREN ARE GRACIOUSLY GIVEN OF GOD. *"The children whom God has graciously given . . ." (Gen. 33:5 KJV).*

"But when it pleased God, who separated me from my mother's womb, and called me by His Grace" (Gal. 1:15 KJV).

*   *   *

End Notes:

[1]   Based on definition from <u>Strong's Greek/Hebrew Dictionary</u>, (Thomas Nelson Publishers) 1984, "vigorous", 2422

CHAPTER SEVEN

DILATION OF CERVIX & NO TEARING

WE MUST CONFESS that God will enlarge us when we need it, just as he tells us to do. As we believe when we pray, we shall have what we say:

> *"Answer me when I call, O God of my righteousness. You have freed me when I was hemmed in and enlarged me when I was in distress; have mercy on me and hear my prayer" (Ps. 4:1 AMP).*

> *"They shall not labor in vain or bring forth (children) for sudden terror or calamity; for they shall be the descendents of the blessed of the Lord, and their offspring with them" (Isaiah 65:23 AMP).*

This is a natural function of the body created by God to do so, just as much as any other natural function of our bodies. Therefore, it should be treated as such – naturally.

AVOID MISCARRIAGE, PREMATURE BIRTH, & BREECH BIRTH.

God promises to fulfill our days. As stated in the Exodus 23 we have:

> *"None shall lose her young by miscarriage or be barren in your land;*
> *I will fulfill the number of your days" (Exodus 23:26 AMP).*

Your baby will come in the perfect timing of God. He said we shall be blessed when we go out. When your baby goes out of your womb it is blessed by Him.

> *"Blessed shall thou be when thou come in, and blessed shall you be when you go out" (Deuteronomy 28:6).*

> *"They shall not labor in vain or bring forth (children) for sudden terror or calamity; for they shall be the descendants of the blessed of the Lord, and their offspring with them" (Isaiah 65:23 AMP).*

> *"Yet You are He Who took me out of the womb; You made me to hope and trust, when I was on my mother's breasts. I was cast upon You from my very birth; from my mother's womb, You are my God" (Psalm 22: 9-10 AMP).*

> *"And the Lord shall make you the head, and not the tail, you shall be above only, and you shall not be underneath" (Deuteronomy 28:13).*

We must depend upon Jesus that when He says He will take our baby from the womb (further described in Chapter Six) that means we will avoid miscarriage, premature birth or breech birth because those types of birth do not line up with what He says He will do. Se we can place our trust in Him to accomplish what He says will be. We can rest assured of a safe delivery.

I always looked at it this way – if this is what the Son of God himself will do for us – then it is either a lie or the truth. Since He is the Son of God – it is the truth and He does not lie. So I place my faith in knowing He will care for me. He tells us to cast our cares upon Him for He cares for us. Need we need anymore?

"Thus says the Lord Who made you and formed you from the womb, Who will help you . . ." (Isaiah 44:2 AMP).

* * *

CHAPTER EIGHT

BLESSINGS OF THE BREAST AND WOMB

OUR FATHER IN Heaven wants to bless his children. It is also part of His Covenant with His children.

> *"By the God of your Father Who will help you, and by the Almighty Who will bless you with the blessing of the heavens above, blessings lying in the deep beneath, of the breasts and of the womb"* (Gen. 49:25 AMP).

> *"Yet You are He who took me out of the womb, You made me hope and trust when I was on my mother's breasts. I was cast upon You from my very birth; from my mother's womb You are my God"* (Psalm 22: 9-10 AMP).

> *"That you may nurse and be satisfied from her consoling breasts; that you may drink deeply and be delighted with the abundance and brightness of her glory"* (Isa. 66:11 AMP).

"And she spoke out with a loud voice, and said "Blessed art thou among women and blessed is the fruit of your womb" (Luke 1:42 KJV).

God shows us by this verse of scripture that it is His desire to bless the fruit of the womb. In Psalms 50:15 he states, "And call on Me . . . I will deliver you." Then in Jeremiah 33:3 AMP He says, *"Call to Me and I will answer you and show you great and mighty things, fenced in and hidden, which you do not know (do not distinguish and recognize, have knowledge of and understand).* He is a God of Abundant Life. All throughout the bible he always heard the prayers of barren women crying out to him to have children. He answered their prayers, sometimes even in the most extreme cases such as Sarah, Hannah, and Elizabeth, Mary's cousin, *(who were all older women). "The Lord listens and heeds when I call to Him" (Ps. 4:3 AMP).* This establishes the fact that He is a God who desires women to conceive regardless of age to fulfill His divine plan for man to multiply upon the face of the earth (Gen. 1:28).

CHILDREN ARE A BLESSING FROM GOD. After I had my daughter I would hold her in my arms and just look at her and look at her. I would thank the Lord for the beautiful gift He had given us. I even began to sing a song to her and the words of which I believe the Holy Spirit gave me. The Word says:

"The children whom God has graciously given" (Gen. 33:5).

"Behold, children are a gift of the Lord:" the fruit of the womb is a reward" (Matt. 18:10).

"As it is written in the Law of the Lord, every (first born) male that opens the womb shall be set apart and dedicated and called holy to the Lord" (Luke 2:23 AMP).

An Inheritance: We have a special inheritance because God also promises to keep His promises to us.

"Know therefore that the Lord thy God, he is God: the faithful God which keepeth covenant and mercy with them that love Him and keep His commandments to a thousand generations" *(Deuteronomy 7:9).*

CHAPTER NINE

ENTERING INTO HIS BLESSING & PEACE

ENTERING INTO HIS BLESSING is what happens when we praise God and confess his word over our life and our baby. God has given us his BLESSING and His PEACE and all we have to do is ask for it. Ask him to give you the peace that passes all understanding that keeps your hearts and minds through Christ Jesus.

Speak this peace and His word over your baby for the blessing. So sing and speak blessings to your child and you can even sing too and you will see God's word and power manifest greatly. It is His will for your life that your baby be the desire of your heart, and a praise to Him. Be bold to come before the throne of grace and ask your Heavenly Father what you desire and he will hear from his holy heaven and answer you.

Another awesome way to bring his peace and calm is through singing praises to him which brings His Presence on the scene. He inhabits the praises of His people. The angels were present and praising when Jesus was born to herald His birth. How much more his own children praising Him, will bring His Glory. I recommend using some great *"anointed" worship* songs and playing them to create an atmosphere of peace. (By anointed, I mean songs that carry the presence of the Holy Spirit on them. You listen to it and you can feel God's presence start to arise upon you and come to you. It is this that breaks every yoke for us. Not all music is anointed even if it sounds good or pretty. It should point in the direction of worship towards His holy heaven and for who He is; for example, He is glorious, He is Wonderful, He is Perfect. It focuses on Him. Check with someone who is a worship leader and they should be able to point you in the right direction.) Because God has given us His peace and all we have to do is ask for it. "Peace I leave with you; My peace I give to you . . ." (John 14:27). Ask him to give you the peace that passes all understanding that keeps your hearts and minds through Christ Jesus. His peace is not as the world gives. He says, "Let not let your heart be troubled, nor let it be fearful" (John 14:27b). Speak this peace and His word over your baby. Your baby is able to hear you after five months.[1] So sing and speak blessings to your child and you will see God's word and power manifest greatly because it is His will for your life that your baby be the desire of your heart and a praise to Him. Be bold to come before the throne of grace and ask your Heavenly Father what you desire and He will hear from His holy heaven and answer you.

The following are some prayers you can say over yourself and your baby:

(*Remember to personalize the pronouns – see italics.*)

> And (*my child*) continues to grow and become strong, increasing in wisdom; and the grace of God is upon *him/ her* (Luke 2:40).

> *My baby will prosper and be in good health, just as (his/her) soul prospers (3 Jn 1:2).*

> The eyes of my baby's understanding are being enlightened; to know what is the hope, calling, and riches of the glory of his/her inheritance in the saints (Eph 1:18 KJV).

My baby is blessed are hungers and thirsts for righteousness, and shall be satisfied (Matt 5:6).

But seek first His kingdom and His righteousness; and all these things shall be added to you (Matt 6:33).

Blessed be the God and Father of our Lord Jesus Christ, who hath blessed us with all spiritual blessings in heavenly places in Christ: (Eph 1:3 KJV).

End Notes:

[1] The Columbia University Complete Guide to Pregnancy, (Crown Publishers, Inc., New York, New York) 1988, 219.

CHAPTER TEN

PRE-NATAL PROFESSIONS

EVERY CHILD IN the womb is subject to what is going on around it in the environment. When a mother speaks negative things such as "I never wanted this baby", or "I need an abortion", she is cursing the child before it even has a chance. Our words are very powerful and we need to watch that what is said around the baby. At this point the mother's professions should be very loving, caring and positive. Many case studies show that babies of mothers who had confessed these negative things had children that were very fretful and irritable as apposed to those who did the opposite – their babies were very calm, quiet and also peaceful. As my own daughter was because of the blessings, good words, and prayers said over her in my womb.

You might think well, can a baby really hear this in the womb. Yes, as we established earlier–they have full auditory capacity at five months, so it is extremely important as to what they are hearing.

Also there can be a lot of emotional wounds from the mother that will be transferred because of the hurts and things that she says. One should watch not to speak these things out. You can ask the Lord to forgive you of anything in your past, to cleanse you and free you from any bondage in the Name of Jesus and you will be able to have peace to pass onto your baby.

The Lord is faithful and just to forgive us of our sins. I John 1.9 says that and he will cleanse us from all unrighteousness as well. Bottom line, stay happy, trusting in the Lord, and be confident that he is able to perform that which perfects us, no matter what.

We know they can perceive what is happening around them as the story of Mary going to visit her cousin, Elizabeth upon greeting Elizabeth it says, the baby leaped in her womb. There was also a promise from God to Zacharias, the father, that His Spirit (the Holy Spirit of God) would be upon the child, "while yet in his mother's womb (Luke 1:15). Zacharias asked how he could be certain and the Angel of the Lord said to him, "I am Gabriel, who stands in the presence of God and I have been sent to speak to you ..." Verse twenty continues with "And behold, you shall be silent and *unable to speak* until the day when these things take place, because you did not believe my words, which shall be fulfilled their proper time.

> "And when he came out, (verse twenty-two), he was unable *to speak* to them and they realized he had seen a vision in the temple" (Luke 1:19-20).

Why was he made to be unable to speak? Because words are powerful–life and death are in the power of the tongue as the scriptures indicate in (Proverbs 18:21) – God did not want Zacharias to negate the promise of a child by any negative words of unbelief, so He was temporarily made mute. Had Zacharias spoke it would have changed everything. Elizabeth then was able to become pregnant–verse 18, even advanced in years. That is the power of our words.

Also significant here is that God has made the husband and/or father the one with God-given authority to speak a blessing or a curse over something. I believe that is why Zacharias had to watch what was coming out of his mouth as the spiritual covering over Elizabeth. So it is very important for father's to speak blessings over their children.

They should lay hands on the womb every day and pray a blessing over their baby for health and protection and peace.

God was answering a man's prayer for a child; sent His Archangel, Gabriel to deliver the message; and blessed them with a son. He will do the same today. He never changes. Hebrews 13.8. Jesus Christ is the same yesterday and today and forever so we can pray a prayer of petition in faith and the Lord will answer according to our faith. Here were two, childless, advanced in years, people who loved God and asked for a child. God answered their prayers. The same for myself, as well. I had to use my faith because of my age. But I had all confidence that all was well and God would peform what He promised me.

You can have the same privilege, as a child of God, to request and it shall be done. Ask him to forgive you of any sins and then pray this scripture: (Mark 11:24) which says, "Therefore I say unto you (Jesus talking), all things for which you pray and ask, believe that you have received them, and they shall be granted you."

Prayer: *Thank you Father, that you forgive me of all my past sins and emotional hurts and give me the peace that passes all understanding that my baby will be perfected by You because as your child and because you formed my child (name the child here) You will sanctify him/her to be emotionally stable, healthy, happy and peaceful, in the name of Jesus Christ.*

CHAPTER ELEVEN

NUTRITIONALLY NURTURED, SPIRITUALLY SOUND

IT IS ALWAYS important to remember that as your baby is, of course, part of you and living in you, it is critical to make sure to have good nutrition for your body. What the mother ingests will be transmitted to the child as the child is feeding from the mother in the womb.

This is just logic. Years ago pregnant women were not advised to watch what they ate or drank, they were probably just told to take some vitamins and even that wasn't so until not too long ago. People really didn't grasp the idea too well that what one does to ones body affects also the fetus in the womb who is growing day by day and forming. It stands to reason if this formation is disturbed or disrupted by unhealthy substances, there will be an affect upon the baby. The baby can be affected spiritually, emotionally, and physically; that is spirit, soul and body.

We already know the baby can hear what is being said about him/her very early on, as I believe I mentioned earlier in the book–they have full auditory capacity at five months. (See Chapter 6, End Notes)

So there is a lot that can be fixed and made correct simply by knowing what the will of God is for your baby. Even though you may have gone through some things don't be discouraged. God loves you and your baby more than you do. He is faithful and just, and will accomplish His Word if we are obedient to use it and pray it.

I encourage you to start using your faith and using the knowledge He has given you as a child of God, to pray over your baby and you will be very happy, and blessed. It doesn't matter what you've been through, just start now praying and holding God to His Word. It is His promise to you.

This isn't a book on nutrition, but I just want to encourage all mothers to get some good *natural* vitamins without preservatives, sugar, artificial colors or flavors added; eat well, eliminate phosphorus-laden sodas and caffeine and you will have a much more peaceful baby. Sugar can be replaced with natural sweeteners such as honey, molasses, Stevia, Agave nectar, etc. Most of all, do *not use* chemical sweeteners of any kind. Avoid junk foods. Eat a lot of vegetables and fruits and protein. At least four or more servings per day. Protein is a great help to building a strong brain and also muscles. Some foods that contain protein are beans, nuts, peanut butter, cheeses, fish, eggs, milk and grass fed meats. Eating three to four servings a day is beneficial. Try to use whole-grain or enriched breads and cereals that do not contain sugar; just add your own sweetener. Again, as logic would dictate, anything with preservatives or chemicals was not designed to go in the body in the first place so why feed it to your new baby. Stick to natural things and nourishing foods and you will, in all probability, see a very bright, alert, healthy baby.

Now that is the physical side of wisdom. However, there is a spiritual side. God gave us a great resource to know what to feed our bodies and our children to help us stay healthy and build our immune systems. But He also lets us know that there is a down side to not listening to his advice. In (Hosea 4:6) it states, *"My people are destroyed for lack of knowledge, and because they have rejected me, I will reject them and their children."*

He loves you and your baby very much and wants the best for you but through lack of knowledge some people create problems for themselves. God wants you to be walking in His kingdom with abundant health and life and He even gives instructions to do so. So grab a hold of His words of wisdom and make them work for you. [See the prayers at the end of the book.]

Granted there are situations where there are certain medical issues, or genetic problems; but a great amount of sickness, illnesses and diseases can be eliminated by being wise with our foods and medicines and then, and also applying spiritual knowledge. There is the hereditary/generational aspect, but that is where God's wisdom comes in again. There are a lot of things one can do in regard to hereditary issues and one of them is by following what the word of God has to say on the subject.

If you said the prayer earlier, then you are a child of God, and if a child then an heir and a child of the promise (Gal. 4:5-7). Therefore, as it says in, (Gal. 3:13 KJV) "Christ redeemed us from the curse of the law, being made a curse for us, for it is written," CURSED IS EVERYONE WHO HANGETH ON A TREE." That wipes out the curses of all generations right there. Jesus took the curses for us. Because we are his covenant children we are redeemed from those curses through Him and His shed blood. We can stand on the word of God and trust that He will bless his children as we use His promises to back it up. We have not because we do not ask. Whatever your history or family generational problems may have been, you can ask Him (the Holy Spirit) to show you what to pray against and loose or bind up and He will show you. "I will give you (Is 22:22; Rev 1:18; 3:7) the keys of the kingdom of heaven; and (Matt 18:18; John 20:23) whatever you bind on earth shall have been bound in heaven, and whatever you loose on earth shall have been loosed in heaven" (Matthew 16:19).

Now, I am not saying you will not have any situations, but what I am saying is that those that you do have can be dealt with on a higher level and changed. All things are subject to change, except the word of God. His word is spirit and truth so what is manifested here on earth had to begin in the spiritual realm first. He is the same yesterday, today and forever. That means we are automatically putting ourselves on the kingdom level of God, using His promise, (the word of the King), to back up what we are praying and believing, and God will back up His own word. He is not a man that he should lie, (Num. 23:19). Jesus said to pray the Father's will be done on earth as it is in heaven, (Matt. 6:9-13). Well in heaven there is no sickness or disease, so we can pray as He instructed and by faith, believe it will happen, and it will because it is not our words but His. Whatever we receive is to be received by faith.

That is, we obtain it by faith, (Matt. 8.10, 13). What He promised He is well-able and faithful to fulfill, (I Cor. 1:9).

PRAYERS FOR MOTHERS-TO-BE

IN THIS SECTION I have put together several prayers for the Mother-to-Be (and the father's as well) to pray over the baby and for themselves. Philippians 4:6 states to be anxious for nothing, but in everything by prayer and supplication with thanksgiving let your **requests** be made **known** to God. So first of all know that God wants to hear your requests and prayers. He wants to answers those prayers. Pray the prayers believing you received them as soon as you have prayed. This is faith, (Mark 11:23). Second, you must be sure that you are a covenant child, which brings the righteousness of God. It means you are entitled to *all* the blessings and promises of God's covenant as a born-again believer.

This is necessary because all the promises of God are based on His righteousness not ours. So, if you are a child of God or if you prayed the prayer in Chapter Two, *His Will and Covenant with You (page 10)*, the good news is that you are the righteousness of God in Christ Jesus and a fellow heir with Christ. Even the righteousness of God which is by faith of Jesus Christ unto all and upon all them that believe: for there is no difference, (Rom. 3:22 KJV). You are in His family and also have the right to come boldly before His throne of grace, making your requests known unto Him (Phil. 4:6), who is able to do exceeding abundantly more than we can ever ask or think. Think of it the same as an earthly father who desires to give anything to his child whom he loves. How much more, your heavenly Father loves you, therefore, he wants to bless you with all heavenly blessings, on earth as it is in heaven (Matt. 6:10).

PRAYERS OF DEDICATION

[You can substitute your baby's name in place of the pronoun, i.e. "you", when you pray this; or you can say to your baby, "*It is written in God's word and I dedicate my child to receive all your blessings that . . .*"]

I thank you Lord that grace and peace be multiplied unto my baby through the knowledge of God, and of Jesus our Lord (2 Pet 1:2 KJV).

You LORD guard our going out and our coming in from this time forth and forever. (Ps 121:8).

For it is God which works in us, both to will and to work for his good pleasure (Phil. 2:13).

PRAYERS TO DECREE A THING

I will decree a thing, and it will be established for me and my baby (Job 22:28).

I speak Your word Lord and it will be, and it will not return to You empty, as it accomplishes what You desire, and succeeds in the matter (Isa. 55:11).

Lord, all things I ask in prayer as I believe I have received I shall receive (Matt. 21:22).

Because my baby is a gift from the Lord, the fruit of my womb is His reward to me (Ps. 127: 3).

My baby and I are strong in the Lord and the power of His might (Eph. 6:10).

We are blessed with all spiritual blessings in heavenly places, in Christ Jesus (Eph. 1:3).

My baby and I will overcome because greater is He that is in me than He that is in the world (1 John 4:4).

As my baby and I become planted in the house of the Lord, we will flourish in the courts of our God (Ps. 92:13).

I will still yield fruit in old age: I shall be fat and flourishing, to show that the Lord is upright (Ps. 92:14).

The Lord will perfect that which concerns me and my baby. (Psalms 138)

It will be done unto me according to my faith (Matt. 9:29).

I will cry to God most high, unto God who performs all things for me (Psalm 57:2).

Lord you bring to pass Your purposes for me and my baby and surely You will complete them.

Lord, you give me and my baby the peace that passes all understanding and guards our hearts and my minds in Christ Jesus (Phil. 4:7).

I am not anxious for anything, but by prayer and supplication and thanks I make my request known to You (Phil. 4:6).

I think and dwell on whatever is true, whatever is honest, whatever is just, whatever is pure, whatever is lovely, whatever is of good report (Phil. 4:8).

Lord, You know the plans you have for me, plans for welfare and not for calamity to give me a future and a hope (Jer. 29:11).

Then I will call upon You and I will come and pray to You and You will listen to me . . . (Jer.29:12).

My baby and I overcame by the blood of the Lamb and the word of my testimony (Rev. 12:11).

PRAYERS OF HIS COVENANT & WILL

I know that You are God, my God; the faithful God which keeps covenant and mercy with them that love Him and keep His commandments to a thousand generations (Deut. 7:9).

For myself and my baby, the Lord my God hath chosen us to be a special people unto himself, above all the people that are upon the face of the earth (Deut. 7:6).

He who began a good work in me and my baby, will continue until the day of Jesus Christ, right up until the time of His return . . . (Phil. 1:6a AMP).

Lord You are developing a good work, and perfecting and bringing it to full completion in us (Phil. 1:6b AMP).

You are at work within us both to will and to do your good pleasure (Phil. 2:13. KJV).

Lord, I call upon You and pray to You, and YouI will listen to me (Jer. 29:12).

I have confidence before You, that, if I ask anything according to Your will You hears me (I John 5:14).

And if we know that He hears us in whatever we ask we know that we have the request which we have asked from Him" (I John 5: 15).

For I know the plans that I have for you, declares the Lord, plans for welfare and not for calamity to give you a future and a hope (Jer. 29: 11).

Then I will call upon You and pray to You, and You will listen to me (Jer. 29:11-12).

He who began a good work in my baby, will continue until the day of Jesus Christ – right up until the time of His return, developing the good work, and perfecting and bringing it to full completion in my baby (Phil. 1:6 AMP).

I confess with my mouth and believe in my heart, the Lord Jesus Christ, and I shall be saved (Acts 16:31).

Lord you said You <u>made</u> me and my baby and <u>formed</u> us from the womb, and You will <u>help</u> us (Isa. 44:2).

Lord Your covenant with me is Your Spirit, Who is upon me and my child and you write Your law inwardly on our hearts . . . (Isa. 59:21a AMP).

Because of Your covenant, Your words which You have put in my mouth shall not depart out of my mouth, or out of the mouth of my [true, spiritual] children, or out of the mouths of my children's children, says the Lord, from henceforth and forever (Isa. 59:21b AMP).

Blessed be the God and Father of our Lord Jesus Christ, who has blessed us with every spiritual blessing in the heavenly places in Christ . . . (Eph. 1:3).

You chose us in Christ <u>before</u> the <u>foundation</u> of the world, that we should be holy and blameless before Him (Eph. 1: 4). (Emphasis added.)

PRAYERS FOR A PERFECT BABY

For You Lord formed my inward parts; You did weave me in my mother's womb (Psalms 139:13).

I will give thanks to Thee, for my baby and I are fearfully and wonderfully made; Wonderful are Thy works, and my soul knows it very well (Psalms 139: 14).

My frame was not hidden from Thee, when I was made in secret, and skillfully wrought in the depths of the earth (Psalms 139: 15).

Your eyes have seen my unformed substance; and in Your book they were all written (Psalms 139: 16a).

I am Your workmanship created in Christ Jesus for good works which God prepared beforehand, that we should walk in them (Eph. 2:10).

Jesus formed my baby, therefore it is positioned properly.

Before You formed me in the belly You Lord knew me; and before I came out of the womb You sanctified me (Jer. 1:5 KJV).

My days were ordained for me, when as yet there was not one of them (Psalms 139: 16c).

For I am confident of this very thing, that You who began a good work in my baby will perfect it until the day of Christ Jesus (Phil. 1:6).

I say You will give us good things (Matt. 7:7,11 KJV).

I decree my baby is perfect, and I have a perfect delivery because Jesus is my deliverer (Psalm 40:17b).

PRAYERS FOR POWER, LOVE & SOUND MIND

For God has not given us a spirit of fear; but of power, and of love, and of a sound mind" (2 Tim. 1:7 KJV).

Christ came and redeemed us from the curse of the law, being made a curse for us (Gal. 3:13).

I command my brain and my body to submit to the word of God and function normally.

I have a sound mind and my baby is sound because of God's wisdom and knowledge.

I shall be preserved through the bearing of children if I continue in faith and love and sanctity with self-restraint (1 Tim. 2:15).

I have life in the power of my tongue; and I love it and shall eat the fruit thereof (Prov. 18:21 KJV).

I observe your commandment and bind them continually on my heart (Prov. 6:20-21).

When I walk about, they will guide me; when I sleep they will watch over me (Prov. 6:22).

When I awake they will talk to me, for your commandment is a lamp, and the teaching is light (Prov. 6:23).

You have given me authority to tread upon serpents and scorpions and over all power of the enemy and nothing shall injure me (Luke 10:19).

Because I fear the Lord and turn away from evil, it will be healing to my body, and refreshment to my bones (Proverbs 3:8).

Your words are life to those who find them, and health to my whole body (Proverbs 4:22).

PRAYERS FOR NO FEAR – NO PAIN

God, You did not give me a spirit of timidity – of cowardice, of craven and cringing and fawning fear – but You have given me a spirit of power, love and a calm and well-balanced mind, discipline, and self-control (2 Tim 1:7 AMP).

<u>Before</u> I travail, I will bring forth; <u>before</u> my pain comes, I will be delivered of my child (Isaiah 66:7 KJV).

I command my body to submit to the Kingdom of God and to function as God created it to, and to have normal muscle contractions.

I will be <u>set securely</u> on high, with long life You will <u>satisfy</u> me (Psalm 91:16 KJV). (Emphasis mine.)

As the uncompromisingly righteous I shall flourish like a palm tree, long-lived, stately, useful, and fruitful (Psalm 92:12 Amp).

I say I am planted in the house of the Lord and I flourish in the courts of my God (Psalm 92: 13).

I will <u>still yield fruit in old age:</u> I shall be <u>full</u> of spiritual vitality and rich in verdure, trust, love and contentment (Psalm 92: 14 AMP).

You said you will contend with him who contends with me, and You will give safety to my children (Isaiah 49:25b Amp).

I come to You, even in weariness, and you give me rest (Matthew 11:28).

I shall find rest for my soul as Your yoke will ease and relieve and refresh (Matthew 11: 28).

For Your yoke is wholesome (useful, good – not harsh, hard, sharp or pressing, but comfortable, gracious and pleasant) and Your burden is light and easy to be borne (Matthew 12:30 AMP).

Christ hath redeemed me from the <u>curse</u> of the law, being made a curse for me (Gal. 3:13 KJV).

For I walk by the law of the Spirit of Life in Christ Jesus which hath made me <u>free</u> from the law of sin and death (Rom. 8:2 KJV).

I have understanding which is a fountain of life unto him that has it (Proverbs 16:22).

PRAYERS FOR SPEEDY PRE-DELIVERY AND SAFE DELIVERY

Because the Hebrew women are <u>not as</u> the Egyptian women; for they are vigorous and <u>they give birth before</u> the midwife can get to them, I will deliver safely and speedily (Exodus 1:19).

I decree that now He is able to do exceeding abundantly beyond all that I ask or think (Eph. 3:20).

I decree that according to the power that works within me, my baby and I shall be delivered, protected, healed, preserved and made whole, if I continue in faith and charity and holiness with sobriety (I Tim. 2:15 KJV).

PRAYERS FOR A FACE-DOWN, HEAD-FIRST DELIVERY

Jesus, you are here to deliver my baby. You will feed Your flock like a shepherd: He shall <u>gather</u> the lambs with <u>Your arms</u>, and <u>carry</u> them in Your bosom, and shall <u>gently lead</u> those that are with young (Isaiah 39:11 KJV).

I decree that before I travail, I will bring forth; <u>before</u> my pain comes, I will give birth with a face-down, head-first delivery (Isaiah 66:7 KJV).

Who has heard such a thing? Who has seen such things" . . . Shall I bring to the point of birth and not give delivery? says the Lord (Isaiah 66:8-9).

You who gives delivery will not shut the womb (Isaiah 66: 9b)?

I declare that Jesus will gather my baby in His arms and carry my child (Isa. 39:11 KJV).

(For averting breech birth)
You Lord, shall make me the head and not the tail, above and not underneath, as I listen to the commandments of the Lord my God (Deut.28:13).

Jesus is my help and deliverer. He will safely deliver my baby (Psalm 40:17b).

I, who have been borne <u>by You from birth</u> and have been <u>carried</u> from the womb . . . You have done it, and You shall <u>carry</u> me and You shall <u>bear me, and You shall deliver me</u> (Isaiah 46: 3-4).

You are He who brings <u>me forth</u> from the womb (Psalm 22:9).

Because I have loved You, therefore <u>You will deliver me</u> (Ps. 91:14).

My child is graciously given by You, Lord (Gen. 33:5 KJV).

It pleased God, who separated me from my mother's womb, and called me by His Grace (Gal. 1:15 KJV).

I am blessed when I come in, and blessed when I go out (Deuteronomy 28:6).

PRAYERS FOR DILATION OF CERVIX & NO TEARING

You have freed me when I was hemmed in and enlarged me when I was in distress (Ps. 4:1 AMP).

I decree I shall not labor in vain or bring forth (children) for sudden terror or calamity; for I shall be the descendents of the blessed of the Lord, and my offspring with them (Isaiah 65:23 AMP).

PRAYERS TO AVOID MISCARRIAGE, AND PREMATURE BIRTH

I shall not lose my young by miscarriage or be barren in my land; You will fulfill the number of my days (Exodus 23:26 AMP).

Lord, You took me out of the womb; You made me to hope and trust, when I was on my mother's breasts (Psalm 22: 9 AMP).

I was cast upon You from my very birth (Psalm 22: 10 AMP).

You, Who made me and formed me and my baby from the womb, You will help me . . . (Isaiah 44:2 AMP).

PRAYERS FOR BLESSINGS OF THE BREAST AND WOMB

God, You will help me, and will bless me with the blessing of the heavens above . . . (Gen. 49:25 AMP).

You God, help me with blessings lying in the deep beneath, of the breasts and of the womb (Gen. 49:25 AMP).

Your blessings upon me will surpass the blessings of my ancestors (Genesis 49:26).

You made me hope and trust when I was on my mother's breasts (Ps. 22.9b).

I was cast upon You from my very birth; from my mother's womb You are my God (Psalm 22: 9-10 AMP).

I decree my baby will nurse and be satisfied from my consoling breasts; that my child may drink deeply and be delighted with abundance (Isa. 66:11 AMP).

I decree I am blessed among women and <u>blessed is the fruit of my womb</u> (Luke 1:42 KJV).

I call to You and You will answer me and show me great and mighty things, fenced in and hidden, which I do not know (do not distinguish and recognize, have knowledge of and understand) (Jer. 33:3 AMP).

Behold, children are a gift of the Lord: the fruit of the womb is a <u>reward</u> (Matt. 18:10).

As it is written in the Law of the Lord, every (first born) male that opens the womb <u>shall be set apart</u> and dedicated and <u>called holy</u> to the Lord (Luke 2:23 AMP).

Know therefore that the Lord thy God, he is God: the <u>faithful God</u> <u>which keeps covenant</u> and mercy with them that love Him and keep His commandments to a thousand generations" (Deuteronomy 7:9).

The Lord listens and heeds when I call to Him (Ps. 4:3 AMP).

PRE-NATAL PROFESSIONS

Jesus you said that all things that I pray and ask, believing I received them, that I shall be granted them (Mark 11:24). So the following are some prayers you can say that will put you in agreement with His Word, therefore you can have faith to believe it will take place because He said to say it. Hallelujah. It is highly significant that the father also pray and speak these blessings over his child to be.

I praise and thank you Lord, that your Spirit would be upon my child yet in my womb (Luke 1:15).

I will watch the words of my mouth that I should not say what I do not want to come to pass.

I thank you Lord, that you are faithful and just to forgive me of all my sins and you will cleanse me from all unrighteousness (1 John 1.9).

ENTERING INTO HIS
BLESSING & PEACE

And my child continues to grow and become strong, increasing in wisdom; and the grace of God (Luke 2:40 NAS).

Beloved, I pray that in all respects my child may prosper and be in good health, just as his/her soul prospers (3 John 1:2 NAS).

The eyes of my child's understanding are being enlightened; that (he/she) may know what is the hope of his/her calling, and what the riches of the glory of his inheritance in the saints (Eph 1:18 KJV).

Blessed are those who hunger and thirst for righteousness, for they shall be satisfied (Matt 5:6 NAS).

I seek first His kingdom and His righteousness; and all these things shall be added to me (Matt 6:33 NAS).

Blessed be the God and Father of our Lord Jesus Christ, who hath blessed us with all spiritual blessings in heavenly places in Christ: (Eph 1:3 KJV).

A Father's Pride & Joy

"My Little Girl was formed
By the Father Most High,
Way before she met her first lullaby.
Her Guardian Angel is ever before His face,
Watching this little one
With love and with grace;
And as she grows in wisdom and beauty,
She won't be alone as she stands –
For her Heavenly Father has her picture
Inscribed on the very palms of His hands."

Matthew 18:10 & Isa 49:16

By C. Brosseau, as inspired by the Holy Spirit

NOTES

www.ingramcontent.com/pod-product-compliance
Lightning Source LLC
Chambersburg PA
CBHW020402290526
45785CB00005B/2409